I0505821

Buried Treasure

A Caregiver's Guide to Unlocking Memories and Creating Happiness

Victoria Jones

Copyright © 2014 Victoria Jones B.A.
All rights reserved.

ISBN: 1507530692
ISBN 13: 9781507530696
Library of Congress Control Number: 2015900581
CreateSpace Independent Publishing Platform
North Charleston, South Carolina

Table of Contents

Introduction

"**UNLESS SOMEONE LIKE** you cares a whole awful lot, nothing is going to get better. It's not."

—Dr. Seuss

This book is about you as the caregiver, intended to help you better understand dementia and develop the knowledge, skills, and passion to walk this journey with your loved one. It will help you not only to provide the best care you can but also to enjoy the special bond that you will share with this person. At the end of the day, I want you to be proud of the care you gave and the special moments you created. These skills will take some time to master, but if you bring passion to this journey, you will both be deeply rewarded. Caregiving is not for sissies, and even people who can handle almost anything may really struggle with the day-to-day needs of a loved one as they progress through the disease. I will give just a little background information on dementia and the stages of Alzheimer's disease just to make sure we are all on the same page.

I have worked in the medical and long-term care (LTC) field for over twenty years, and the level of our understanding and the culture of care have changed dramatically in that time. In the old days, we would focus on "reality orientation"—trying to keep a woman with memory loss in the moment by constantly reminding her of things she had forgotten. This was not only fruitless but cruel as well, as the common practice, for example, was to remind her that her spouse had died when she asked about him, thus causing widows to grieve all over again. We have since learned that "joining the journey" or going along with the participants in their questions made it not only easier to get them redirected but also much less traumatic. I will share examples with you throughout this book to help you with redirection and fibbing, as these can be difficult to master when you have a long history of believing that truth is always most important! This book is a quick once-through read. You can go back as needed and reread sections when new issues arise. My goal is to convey a lot of information in a short space, as busy caretakers won't have time to read a long book. I hope you find this guide helpful.

I used female pronouns throughout the book primarily to avoid having to write "him or her" and to be consistent. According to the Alzheimer's Association, a woman's risk of developing Alzheimer's after age 65 is 1 in 6, a man's risk is 1 in 11.

I also refer to the person with dementia as "the participant" as that is the term we use in the Adult Day Care industry and it seems less clinical than "patient".

1
What Is Dementia?

DEMENTIA IS THE umbrella term for "altered mental status." This can include many things and can be temporary or permanent. Dementia is *not* a normal part of aging; however, as we age, the percentage of people in our cohort with dementia increases. A medication or infection can cause temporary dementia symptoms that disappear when the medication is stopped or the infection is cleared up. If the memory loss and confusion occurs suddenly, a full medical workup is needed to determine its cause. In this book we are talking of ongoing memory loss or confusion.

Alzheimer's disease is the most common form of dementia, accounting for about 70 percent of those with dementia. Alzheimer's is progressive and ultimately fatal, with an average life expectancy of seven to ten years after diagnosis. The brain actually shrinks as the disease progresses, which can be seen in an MRI, and brain signals are not sent correctly to the other parts of the body to maintain all body function. Over time, the body shuts down. It seems to me that folks who are diagnosed before the age of sixty-five have a faster decline than those who are diagnosed in later years. That is a long journey for an illness, not only for the participant but also for everyone around her. From the first day of diagnosis, life will never be the same. If your loved one has been diagnosed or if you suspect Alzheimer's disease, visit a specialist, get her checked out, and discuss a course of treatment. There are some medications and lifestyle changes that can help slow its progression. Include your loved one in the decisions early on, as you will need to get her affairs in order while she is still competent.

Call a family meeting and get everyone involved. *Do not try to handle this alone!* Remember how Hillary Clinton said many years ago that "it takes a village to raise a child"? Well, it takes a village to care for a senior with Alzheimer's disease as well. Get commitments early on from family, friends, neighbors, churchgoers, and club members your loved one knows. The more people looking out for her, the better.

What is Sundowning?

Generally it is increased anxiety or agitation occurring primarily in the late afternoon or evening, often worsened by fatigue.

2

Stages of Alzheimer's Disease

STAGE 1: IN this stage she will suffer minimal lapses in memory that could also be attributed to normal aging.

Stage 2: The sufferer may notice lapses in memory and utilize notes and other cues to compensate. Others may not detect those lapses, and a medical exam would likely not reveal a problem.

Stage 3: Symptoms may include difficulty recalling names or words; difficulty at work, such as forgetting recent assignments; difficulty in social settings; misplacing objects more often than usual or putting them in unusual places; forgetting what has just been read; and difficulty in planning a multistep project. Family, friends, and coworkers may notice a decline in memory and communication. A medical examination is likely to diagnose MCI (mild cognitive impairment) or early AD (Alzheimer's disease). Symptoms can still be missed at this stage by family and friends, even more so if the participant is married. Often spouses cover for each other, sometimes unknowingly, by finishing sentences for each other or not bothering to complete thoughts, as the other person knows what is meant. When others notice this, it has probably been going on for years, and they do not realize that it has gotten more pronounced. Since this is very typical between couples, it is important that if you suspect dementia, you'll need to spend a few hours alone with your loved one without the interference or "help" from her spouse to obtain a sense of how significant the memory issues may be.

Stage 4: Social withdrawal is more prevalent, as the person fears making mistakes and has decreased ability to organize and plan, difficulty with finances and math, difficulty performing complex tasks, and less recall of recent events or social engagements. Depression also may be more obvious. She may seem more compliant, as she is looking to someone else to make decisions she then goes along with. I often call this "pleasantly confused," as she may not know what to do but is happy to do what is suggested. She may start an activity and keep going for hours because she is very proud of herself when she makes progress on a craft or jigsaw puzzle, and may not initiate a new activity without encouragement from someone else.

Stage 5: Impairments are more noticeable, even to strangers. She may have difficulty keeping track of time and place but still be able to remember her own name and names of significant family members or long-term friends. Judgment is impaired; however, she can likely still eat and use the bathroom without assistance. Upon medical examination, she is likely diagnosed with moderate AD.

Stage 6: She will have difficulty recognizing spouse and close family members, behavioral and personality changes, reduced awareness of surroundings, more difficulty communicating and understanding the meaning or use of objects, need for prompting or cuing with almost all tasks, significant memory decline, bowel and bladder incontinence, and more prevalent psychiatric symptoms mark this stage.

Stage 7: This final stage is marked by the need for total assistance in daily living, difficulty understanding surroundings, impaired swallowing, impaired motor coordination, being wheelchair or bed bound, and impaired basic communication. Upon medical examination, the patient is likely diagnosed with advanced AD.

3

Deny/Delay/Change the Subject/Make Excuses

YOUR INTENTIONS WERE good. You took Mom to the doctor, and he confirmed your suspicions, but now the family doesn't share your concerns. You think it is so obvious; why are they arguing with you? It takes time for news like this to sink in. To family members who live out of town or only see Mom for a couple of hours a week, she may seem totally normal. Everyone forgets things, right? You see her every day and have noticed that she is forgetting things and making serious mistakes with her bills, so how can you both be right?

Denial is the most common response when we first hear that a loved one may have dementia. This is understandable. We don't want to face that diagnosis. We don't want to overreact and misinterpret a little forgetfulness, or most significantly, we just don't want it to be true. All are very understandable reasons to deny the diagnosis. The most important thing is to listen to family and friends who also care about your loved one and then educate yourself. Get help early, and talk to your siblings or other family members regularly to keep track of how things are going and to keep everyone on the same page.

Picture yourself getting ready for a job interview. You are going over the points in your mind that you want to make. You go over how you will answer the anticipated questions so you sound confident in your answers, and then you hardly sleep the night before because you are so nervous. That is the way your mom is handling your visiting sibling. She is doing mental gymnastics to prepare, and her occasionally evasive answers go unnoticed. At the restaurant, she orders from a picture or just tells the server to give her the same thing as someone else to avoid making a decision. She is covering up; after a two- or three-hour visit, she is exhausted, and her visitors leave convinced that all is well.

4

Typical Day Alone

IMAGINE THAT YOU fall asleep and wake up some years later, as if you've been caught in a time warp. You look around, and things look somewhat familiar, but it just doesn't feel right. The neighbor comes by to visit, and you recognize her, but she is talking of events and people you cannot recall. She asks you questions that you realize you should know the answer to, so to avoid looking stupid, you are evasive with your answers. This seems to satisfy her, so you go along. If she asks too many questions, you get anxious because you don't want to let on that you don't know; however, if she keeps chattering away, you are more than happy to just listen.

After a few minutes, she hands you a casserole dish for your dinner, and you graciously thank her and put it in the refrigerator. She bids you farewell, and you decide it is a good time for a nap. Soon after, you are awakened by a phone call. The friendly voice on the other end of the line exchanges pleasantries and lets you know that the local politician is counting on your support again this November and could really use a financial contribution as well. You realize that you must know her, so you get out the credit card and give her all the information she may need to process your contribution because they need your help. She then invites you to a fund raiser, which you accept because you are so looking forward to seeing the candidate again on Friday.

After hanging up, you realize that the mail has come, so you trot out to the mailbox to collect it. There are many envelopes and bills. Some are for utilities, and many are asking for contributions. They all say, "Act Now," so you comply and write checks for all of them and put them back out in the mail. You don't really know what you should be doing next, but you decide to organize the drawers of your dresser, as you can't seem to find the clothes that you wanted to wear today. You start some laundry in the basement but get sidetracked throughout the day and never get back to it. The clothes you emptied and stacked from the dresser remain on the bed. You turn on the television and are frightened by the amount of violence in the world. That's odd; none of the newscasters look familiar. Then an infomercial comes on and tells you how much this new gadget will save you in time and trouble, and you decide to get it, not sure how you ever lived without it. You again dig out the credit card and make the purchase. The friendly voice on the other end of the line lets you know of several other special offers, and you think you called on a very lucky day!

After another short nap, your granddaughter calls to check on you. "What did you do today?" she asks. You let her know you were very busy handling this and that. She reminds you that you have a doctor appointment in the morning and that she will pick you up at nine o'clock. You hang up the phone and again turn the TV on. The evening wears on—the casserole forgotten, laundry not finished, several credit transactions forgotten, checks written without worry whether there were funds available—and you fall into a troubled slumber. Your stomach is empty, and your body is not worn out in the least, as you had so little physical activity today. Medications remain in the bottle as you finally drift off. When the doorbell rings at nine o'clock the next morning, you stumble to answer it, only to see a stranger standing on your doorstep.

Ouch! How does that feel? Did you notice that you struggled a little more when you were first awakened and did better once you had a chance to listen for a little bit? Did you notice that the TV caused more anxiety than it helped alleviate? Did you notice how vulnerable you would be to an unscrupulous person who wanted to take advantage? This example probably describes someone in stage 3 or early stage 4 of the disease. Both the granddaughter and the neighbor are involved, and with just a little more support and some meaningful activities for the day, the day would be so much more fulfilling.

To really experience something, you must use all of your senses to be fully engulfed in all it has to offer. For example, as a child I enjoyed summer evenings without a care in the world. I relive that experience now by taking off my shoes in the cool grass and wiggling my toes, listening to the locusts, smelling the freshly cut grass, and watching the sun set. No matter what has happened that day, taking a few minutes and immersing myself in that experience provides a relaxing, calming end to my day. When I come back inside, I am that carefree child of eight again.

You have probably had similar experiences or reminders of good times. While you are thinking about them, take the time to close your eyes and remember the smells, sensations, and sounds, and just imagine yourself again immersed with all of your senses. It will be much more powerful!

5

What Is Happiness?

ACCORDING TO DR. Martin Seligman, past president of the American Psychological Association, there are five factors that contribute to happiness: positive emotion and pleasure, achievement, relationships, engagement, and meaning. You will see these factors interwoven into the foundations of care immersion. When caregiver and participant are both engaged in meaningful interactions and focused on positive emotions and experiences, both will have a good day and not just a day full of the tasks of caring for another.

"Live with intention. Walk to the edge. Listen hard. Practice wellness. Play with abandon. Laugh. Choose with no regrets. Appreciate your friends. Continue to learn. Do what you love. Live as if this is all there is."

—Dr. Seuss

6

The Dense Fog of a Caregiver

THIS SOUNDS WEIRD, but let me explain. When a mother brings home a newborn, she experiences sleep deprivation, a steep learning curve, and lack of personal time. This phase is generally short lived; the baby begins sleeping more at night, the routine is evened out, and the new mom learns how to adapt her schedule. Life never goes back to where it was, but she finds a new normal, and the joy of the little one outweighs any personal sacrifice she has to make.

Caring for an elder, especially one with dementia, is harder, partly because it can last so much longer and because the care needs usually increase over time.

In foggy conditions, you must turn on your headlights, but the bright headlights make it harder to see. You can only see a short distance in front of you; you cannot see the path ahead of you in order to decide which way to go at the fork until you are there. Hence, you cannot really plan because you are just driving through this fog on a road that you don't know. How do you know if you are in the fog? Do you see yourself in the descriptions below?

- You have nice clothes but no accessories.
- Your hair is nice, but the style is grown out.

- You wear very little or no makeup.
- You are sleep deprived.
- You do not easily engage in conversation with strangers, or you appear self-absorbed.
- You shop strictly from a list and do not read labels.
- You are often in a rush.
- You are no longer involved in community, church, or social activities.
- You have withdrawn from hobbies, such as hunting, fishing, sewing, golfing, tennis, etc.
- You ignore all but most crucial medical appointments for yourself.
- You are no longer involved in any structured exercise.
- You are no longer involved in volunteer or charity work.
- Your house needs repairs and maintenance.
- Your car needs maintenance.
- Your total frame of reference for any conversation revolves around the care recipient.
- Your friends and family have stopped calling.
- You think that no one can do the job that you are doing.

No judging here—I'm just trying to help you see that you deserve to have a full life, which may include caregiving, but not at the expense of everything else.

Obviously, if you make the commitment to be a full-time caregiver, your schedule and personal time will change, but what I really want to convey in this book is that losing yourself to the caregiving tasks serves no purpose. You will become enveloped in the dense fog and alienate those around you who would be delighted to help if only you would let them in to take on a few tasks every month to lighten your load. I have yet to meet a caregiver who has even scratched the surface of utilizing the resources that are available to help. You can be an excellent caregiver and still maintain the important other parts of your life and escape the enveloping fog.

The solution is the streetcar analogy.
Let's imagine the participant is riding on a streetcar powered by steam. The streetcar follows a set path; you will get on for periods of time and off for periods of time. You will let others get on the streetcar with her regularly, and you will find destinations along the way at which you can reminisce and enhance her experiences. You will have created an environment on the streetcar that keeps her safe so that she does not require your undivided attention, and you will have loaded the streetcar with things she finds engaging.

This is how you keep your sense of self, honor the other people in your life, and most of all, know at the end of the day that you made good decisions so you can be guilt-free. You will be able to see the path ahead clearly and make decisions at each station instead of aimlessly driving through the fog.

Here are ten foundations to help you stock and run your streetcar:

1. Provide a supportive environment in which the participant has the freedom to roam, touch, organize, rearrange, and otherwise do as she pleases.
2. Utilize cues to assist in successful completion of tasks.
3. Utilize sensory stimulation and music to enhance full engagement and reduce anxiety.
4. Provide meaningful activities throughout the day for cognitive and physical stimulation.
5. Structure the day to accommodate the participant's natural rhythm, once it is found, and keep the same structure each and every day.
6. Only ask questions that engage the participant, not needless questions that test her memory (e.g., "What did you have for lunch?"). Also, take the word "no" out of your vocabulary. When that word is needed, redirect instead.
7. Provide opportunities every day to share successes and reminisce about happy times. Seek her advice when appropriate and ask for her help.

8. Provide regular opportunities to contribute to others (e.g., volunteering at the local animal shelter or taking the newspaper to the shut-in next door).
9. Ensure that personal care is attended to by providing the cues and assistance needed while maintaining as much independence as possible, never stealing her dignity.
10. Keep a sense of humor!

This may seem a little overwhelming at first, but let's break it down into manageable chunks. Since the streetcar can be powered by steam, we need to raise it to 212 degrees in order to create steam. At 211 degrees the water is only hot and will not provide the needed power; you will have to. Let's assume for a moment that your spouse has recently been diagnosed with dementia, and you have decided to be the primary caregiver, so you are reading this book for some help. Fantastic! The fact that you realize that there may be more to it than you currently understand means that you are a model student.

Let's also assume that your caregiving up until now has been to remind your spouse to take her medications and make sure she gets to the doctor. At this point your caregiving skills would be at room temperature—let's say 72 degrees. You are making sure that she remembers to do things, but that has been the extent of it so far. You now realize how valuable these experiences will be and decide you want to put her on the streetcar and use steam to help power it. To do that, you need to step up the temperature by 140 degrees. Until then you will be providing all the power by sheer force, but once you reach that magic number, the streetcar will start coasting along. Each evening take a few minutes to reflect on how the day went—your loved one's level of engagement, activities you did together, her level of anxiety, the amount of sleep she needed, and so forth. Think of one thing you can improve upon for the next day and write it down.

You will make mistakes, and you will have bad days, so just realize that up front. You must fail or stick your foot in your mouth to have success tomorrow; it's just the way it works. In exactly 140 days, or less than five months, you will have increased the heat to 212 degrees if you follow this systematic approach. You will still have difficulties, and each time your loved one has another decline, you will readjust some things you are doing. That's why keeping a journal is crucial. You can identify patterns and quickly establish a new routine. Your stories and methods for redirecting will chug along because it doesn't take much energy to keep the water simmering!

The streetcar analogy really focuses on participants in stages 4 through 7. If your loved one is in stage 3, my advice is to take that trip you have always wanted to go on or visit out-of-town family members while you still can and can really enjoy it together. Just remember to allow extra time each day for rest and try to not to plan too much stimulation.

Also take the time now to discuss her wishes for later, when she may not be able to communicate them to you. Each of you should complete a document such as Caring Conversations, available from the Center for Practical Bioethics and free to download from their website. It can also be ordered for three dollars if you prefer the printed version. This is a good way to start conversations with our loved ones to learn what their wishes are and how we can fulfill them. Focus on eating right, exercising, getting fresh air, and enjoying every moment. For the participant in stages 4 and 5, you will see the most benefit from implementing these foundations, and this will carry you forward into the later stages very well.

"Today was good. Today was fun. Tomorrow is another one."

—Dr. Seuss

7

Ten Foundations Explained

Provide a supportive environment in which the participant has the freedom to roam, touch, organize, rearrange, and otherwise do as she pleases.

TAKE A WEEKEND to declutter and babyproof your house. If you have a lot of knickknacks sitting around, thin them out. Remove area rugs and put all cleaning supplies or hazardous chemicals out of easy reach. You want to have the room set up so that if she is there by herself you do not have to supervise. You know she is safe. If you have priceless possessions, start packing them away. There will likely come a time when your loved one is fiddling, packing, and rearranging everything within reach, and you don't want to be sitting on pins and needles hoping your priceless trophy does not fall to the floor and shatter! You will want to keep photos and perhaps a scrapbook or memory book on the coffee table for easy access.

Let's focus on the living room. Once you have decluttered it, the next step is to place a few memory or project stations throughout the room. I have a list of these in the appendix; use the ones you feel are most appropriate for your situation, four to six of them, depending on her needs. If your loved one is very busy, you will likely want six. You want things that she can investigate by herself when you are otherwise engaged. You can also use these stations for a task that you start together but that she will continue on her own while you leave for a few minutes to make a phone call or do some similar task. Be sure to provide positive feedback and show your appreciation when she completes a task.

Eventually you may need at least a couple of project stations in each room. For example, the dining room is a good place to always have a jigsaw puzzle going on the table and maybe a basket of socks to sort nearby.

To be safe, the environment must be secure. If your loved one opens a door, you will want to know whether it is to leave or to let someone in. If your house has an alarm system, you can set it to sound a beep each time the door is opened. If you don't have an alarm, you can buy an inexpensive wireless one for each door at Radio Shack or another electronic store. At this point this should be sufficient, unless she is actively trying to leave. I will discuss "exit-seeking" behavior in a later section. You may assume that your loved one will never wander or try to leave because she is home. Roughly half the folks with AD wander. The thing is, I don't think they are necessarily trying to leave; they just go outside for a valid reason and get side-tracked. If they wander around outside for a long time, they may forget their way back. You just don't know if or when this may happen, so you need to take some precautions early on. If she begins to wander, then be very aggressive in your safety precautions.

A significant number of folks will pack, unpack, organize, wrap, and otherwise busy themselves for no apparent reason. Just let her do it as long as she is not overly anxious. She is trying to accomplish something, so let her have that. You can always put things back later if you need to. Take a deep breath, and don't worry about it.

Staff at a local memory care unit found that their residents were not receptive to the project stations they had set up. The participants had been very affluent and did not usually perform those tasks, as they'd had maids and cooks to do them. The staff got creative and turned one activity room into a boutique and the dining area into a club. Each day the ladies would shop at the boutique and have lunch at the club. They worked on their golf swings with their "pro" and often went to the spa or salon. They would take their purchases to their "suites," and later in the evening, the staff would retrieve the clothes and return them to the boutique for another day of shopping. Buried treasure! I love this term because it reflects the perfect connection with the participant's true self and their memories, relationships or environment. These opportunities can happen accidentally, but as you develop your skills, you will be better able to find these treasures in your everyday interactions with your loved one.

The day's activities must be reflective of how she spent her days to be meaningful. Just filling the days with items on the calendar is not enough.

Utilize cues to assist in successful completion of tasks.
There are many types of cues: verbal, written, physical, and visual. Starting with stage 4, you will likely see that the participant has less concern with personal care and hygiene. Once reminded to do the task, she may be willing to do it but does not realize that it needs to be done in the first place. She may be hesitant to shower and change clothes, layer her clothes, and forget to brush her teeth or not do it properly. Initially a note taped to the bathroom mirror may be sufficient to remind her to wash her face, brush her teeth, and comb her hair. Laying the items out in the order needed would also help by providing a visual cue of what implement to use; this can help maintain her

independence. Later you will need to provide hands-on cuing or step-by-step instructions to get the task done.

Initially, starting the shower and laying out the soap and shampoo will get the ball rolling, but later you may need to be more insistent. We'll discuss that in a later segment. Since changing clothes can be an obstacle with many folks, use the time that she is in the shower to gather all of the dirty clothes and take them to the laundry room—where they will be out of sight and out of mind—and lay out clean clothes for her to put on. Many folks will hang up their clothes and then put them on again the next day, so even if they are showering regularly, the clothes take on a life of their own. If you get into the habit of removing the clothes now, it will be less of an issue later.

As long as your loved one is continent, don't worry too much about reminders to use the bathroom except before leaving the house or going to bed.

A calendar is an important cue that we all use. It is especially helpful in stages 2 through 4. I like to use one that is a little larger than average and attaches magnetically to the refrigerator. Mark off the days that have passed, and plan your week in advance by putting four to six things on the calendar each day. Of course you would list any appointments, but also add things that you plan to do together. If you are going to the park on Wednesday to feed the ducks, put it on there; if you are going to a grandson's ball game, put it on the calendar. This will help remind her of upcoming events and give her more of an opportunity to think about and look forward to them. When she sees a full day of activities planned, it's easier to get her motivated to get going.

Wherever your calendar is, hang some pictures nearby. Use a collage-type frame and include all of the family members either individually or in small groups (e.g., daughter and her husband in one photo, two grandsons in the other). If the participant is starting to struggle to remember names, go ahead and label the photos. Don't make her struggle. Since long-term memories are more vivid, you may also want to include pictures from thirty to fifty years ago of many of those same people.

Beside each telephone, you'll want a pad of paper and a pen so if she answers the phone she can write down a note. It may also be helpful to put a reminder there to not give any personal information over the phone. This may help if you get a lot of sales calls; see the section on handling money issues. If she spends any time alone, you may want to put a note on the inside of the front door reminding her to look out the window before opening the door to make sure she knows who is calling.

If you want her to come with you, but she doesn't understand, use hand signals along with the words "please come" or "let's go." You are giving her two opportunities to understand your message: verbal and visual. You can also use pictures for your bathroom cue cards if she no longer understands the tasks she should be doing, such as brushing her teeth and washing her face. You could see how she responds to a list on the bathroom mirror using pictures of the toothbrush and washcloth.

An example of a physical cue is touching a part of the body while you are talking about it, or touching the chair you are asking her to sit down in. This is most effective if she sometimes calls a familiar item by the wrong name or doesn't understand your simple message. It may be that the wire is just crossed in her brain; when you point to the chair or pat the seat, she knows what you want her to do.

Utilize sensory stimulation and music to enhance full engagement and reduce anxiety.
You can provide sensory stimulation with scents using sachets, candles, sprays, scented wax cubes, and a whole host of other options. Lavender helps people sleep, so a little spray on sheets

or a sachet in the pajama drawer could really help. I like to vary scents throughout the day so they are fresh and the brain doesn't get used to them. One place I worked, we made a loaf of bread every day in the bread machine. We started it at exactly 10:00 a.m. so that the aroma was fabulous at noon when we were gathering everyone for lunch. We would ask the residents if they could smell the bread and comment on how wonderful it was. Often they would start filing down to the dining room on their own without being reminded. Even with their memory loss, by tying the aroma to a desired action, the brain often made a connection. Food smells also help to stimulate appetite. As you smell food, your brain realizes you are hungry, and your digestive juices start working, thus increasing appetite. Often a person with dementia will not be hungry until she actually smells the food, so just asking if she is hungry will almost always result in a no.

Utilizing scents of favorite foods, like apple pie, often promotes a happy feeling. Try pumpkin spice in the fall, apple cider, vanilla, or coffee. These can all be individualized to your loved one.

Music is also very powerful in increasing engagement. Music is processed in a different area of the brain than words. I like to use favorite music from different eras of participants' lives, but you can also use upbeat music in the morning and softer, calmer music in the evening. See what she responds best to, but just remember that if she is hard of hearing, you may need to have the music a little louder than you would actually like. If she liked to dance when she was younger, ask her what music she danced to and use it when you want to dance. How can you dance and not be transported to a happy time? Music triggers memories, which trigger positive responses, which will open up many opportunities for positive reminiscing and bringing it all together. If you know how to create a playlist on an MP3 player, about forty songs will probably be enough.

As she progresses and has more difficulty understanding your words, sometimes singing the instructions can help her to understand. For instance, after a shower, when you are trying to dry each part of her body, you might sing the "Hokey Pokey": "You put your right foot in; you put your right foot out. You put your right foot in, and you shake it all about." If you can condense that a little, she may respond very well to the instructions.

When walking with someone who is having difficulty even remembering to put one foot in front of the other, I often sing the "left, left, left, right, left" cadence and just keep going with it. Almost every time her brain will kick in and she starts walking in time with my silly song. My other two favorites are "These Boots Are Made for Walking" and "Walking on Sunshine." Both work well when motivating participants to walk with me, either to get away from something that is causing them anxiety or to just build some rapport if they are upset. Both songs will reduce anxiety almost immediately, and you will likely be laughing together in a minute or two. Be a little silly, and don't be afraid to make fun of yourself. In turn, she will let her guard down and laugh at herself as well.

At our center, we use the Pandora spa station app to play music in the front area. The music is relaxing, and sometimes a participant will hover there if she's anxious about being at the center or wants to go home. Usually after fifteen or twenty minutes of hearing the music and with staff helping to calm her the anxiety, she is ready to engage in an activity. I've tried it without music, but it is much harder and takes longer, so now the music comes on automatically in the morning. It may also help family members dropping people off, as they feel a sense of calm as well.

We also have a nice fragrance in the front area. I like scents like rain or aloe—not really like perfume, just a freshness that awakens the senses.

Provide meaningful activities throughout the day for cognitive and physical stimulation.

In order for both of you to have a good day, you can't leave it to chance. You must plan. You will need a large calendar that you can fill with any appointments, activities that you can do together, and mementos. You will also need a place, such as a journal, to document your "one degree" of improvement each day to keep yourself accountable.

There are hundreds of activities that you and your loved one can do together, things that challenge her some but that she can be successful at. You will also want age-appropriate materials and not games or puzzles that are too juvenile. If your spouse likes to cook or bake, this is very valuable time you can spend together, with you providing minimal cuing and oversight and her taking the spatula, so to speak, and running with it. Instead of buying a cake from the store for the church potluck on Sunday, bake one on Saturday afternoon. She may really enjoy selecting the recipe, helping you gather the ingredients, measuring and stirring them, and smelling the wonderful aroma as it bakes. She will be so proud to have contributed. Make sure everyone knows that she baked the cake so when they have a piece so they can compliment her. You needed to keep her busy for the afternoon, and she needed to be needed, so it's a win-win situation for you both.

In the earlier stages of the disease, she may do very well following a recipe to make something from scratch; you may need to help with reading the recipe and measuring the ingredients, but she may do fine with the rest. Later, you may need to use a cake or cookie mix and measure the ingredients and then let her stir it. Either way, it is a meaningful activity that serves many needs.

Yard work and fixing things are just as important in filling the day. Your loved one may no longer be able to mow the grass but could rake leaves, weed the flower bed, or water the garden. It may seem like a project that should take two hours, but it can be spread out as busy work for days if needed. Laundry is similar. Socks can be sorted, resorted, and matched again several times a day. Whichever tasks your loved one gravitates to, give her many opportunities to complete them. You don't want her to feel as though she has so much work to do that she will never get it done; it should be just enough for her to feel that she has things she can do most of the day.

Structure the day to accommodate the participant's natural rhythm, once it is found, and keep the same structure each and every day.

A day may look something like this:

7:30 a.m.	Wake up and personal care
8:00 a.m.	Breakfast and review calendar for the day's activities
8:45 a.m.	Do the dishes and tidy the house—one or two chores each day
9:30 a.m.	Exercise—either following a DVD or doing something outside
10:30 a.m.	Cognitive activity
11:30 a.m.	Organizing activity at the table, such as clipping coupons, sorting socks, looking at a cook book, or doing a puzzle
12:00 p.m.	Lunch
1:00 p.m.	Run errands, take a walk, or do something physical
2:30 p.m.	Quiet time to take a nap or listen to music
4:00 p.m.	Bake or do yard work—keeping busy at this time usually reduces sundowning
5:30–7:00 p.m.	Dinner, dishes, and dog walking
7:00 p.m.	Dial it down by listening to music, reading a book to her, or watching an old movie on TV
8:30 p.m.	Prepare for sleep; lower the lights in the house

It may take two or three times longer for personal care tasks and eating than it used to, so plan plenty of time for those when you have a schedule to keep. If the above routine is similar to yours, then you would never make a doctor appointment for 9:00 a.m., as you likely wouldn't be able to make it. You would want to make it for 10:30 a.m. or later in the morning; otherwise, you may be too rushed. If the appointment needed to be in the afternoon, something around 1:30 p.m. would be perfect. If it needs to be later, you may want to make sure you take something to the appointment that she can work on to avoid the anxiety or boredom that often comes up later in the afternoon.

Keep a tote bag packed with crosswords, word-search books, lace cards, craft projects, puzzles, sorting games, and so forth, either by your front door or in your car, for just such occasions. You may still be able to attend community meetings, church activities, and short community events with her; just make sure she has something to focus on if the event goes on long enough for her to get bored or anxious.

Only Ask Questions That Engage the Participant, Not Needless Questions That Test Her Memory (e.g., "What did you have for lunch?"). Also, Take the Word "No" Out of Your Vocabulary. When That Word Is Needed, Redirect Instead.
If you are not with your loved one all the time, then you may be tempted to start a conversation by asking an open-ended question, such as "What did you have for lunch?" You may think this a good conversation starter, and it would be in other circumstances, but not for the person with dementia. She is immediately embarrassed because she doesn't remember what she had and is angry with you for making her feel that way. It is critically important to remember when dealing with anyone, but especially someone with dementia, that while she may not always remember you, she

will always remember how you made her feel. She will lash out at you if she thinks that you make her feel stupid.

Asking more questions in an effort to pry the answer out of her will only make things worse. Throw out all those general conversation starters and use soft-serve starters instead. How about: "I know Mary took you out to Mel's Diner for meatloaf today. Was it as wonderful as always?" If you don't know what they ate, focus on the visit she had with Mary. "Did you and Mary have a wonderful time at lunch today?" She may not remember the actual lunch, but you gave her some content to work with in answering you. You want to soft serve the questions and give her many directions in which to go with her answers. She may focus on how wonderful Mary is, the diner as her favorite place to eat, or how wonderful the meatloaf is, and then take the conversation from there.

While on the subject of asking and answering questions, here are two difficult topics that will likely come up and how to address them.

"I Want to Go Home"

Home is a feeling, not an address. Many folks will talk about going home even though they have lived in the same house for fifty years, so there is no other explanation than that it is not the address but a place that feels safe. Often when a participant has moved to a long-term care facility, she will speak of going home. Everyone assumes that home is the place she just moved from and tells her that she can no longer live alone, that the staff is there to help her, and so on. They think this is good information to share, but that is not at all what the participant needs. She needs to *feel* like she is at home.

Think about the things that have made you feel safe over the years, and implement those same things in your response. "Tell me about your home. Who lives there with you? When you go outside, what do you see?" She may tell you that she sees the lake with the ducks, and you can then discuss how much you enjoy the lake and feeding the ducks. She may say that she lives there with her parents and three siblings, and you can then ask what kind of work her father did or what chores she is supposed to do when she gets home from school. When you go this direction with your response, you will have numerous areas in which to take the conversation other than, "No, you can't go home. You live here now."

For spouses this can be especially troubling because she may realize that she has a husband named John but does not associate the man with her as her husband, as he is *old!* She remembers John as a young man, so if she is distraught about going home to her husband, instead of telling her that John is her husband, which will only scare her half to death, ask her to tell you about John. Show her a picture of John as a young groom, and see how she responds. Most likely she will talk lovingly of him when seeing the picture, and then you can tell her that John is much older now. Show her a picture of John as an older man, and perhaps this will reduce her fear. Then when she actually looks at John, she may connect for a moment. Buried treasure!

The second topic that can be difficult is when a participant asks about someone who has died. Sometimes in the earlier stages of the disease, we can just remind her that someone passed away. If it is not a close relative, the reminder is not upsetting. But for any close family members, stick with redirecting. Here's an example: "I need to get home; my mother is looking for me." Perhaps the mother passed many years ago, and you are surprised by this statement. Your first tendency would be to tell her that her mother is dead, but you now know this is not the right approach. So what do you do? Some examples of redirection follow. Some will not work, but others will work well. You just have to experiment, because you can guarantee that you will get many opportunities to perfect this skill!

"Does your mother need you to help her with something? How about we make some cookies until we hear from her?"

"I haven't talked to her today, but I talked to your husband, and he made arrangements for you to eat lunch with us today. Your husband is so sweet. You are so lucky to have such a wonderful man!"

"I don't think your mother is at home, but what can we do today to help her?"

The participant needs to feel that she is doing what she should be doing today because she feels out of sorts, so once you address that feeling and give her something to do that makes sense to her, you will reduce her anxiety. Around three or four in the afternoon, sundowning is at its worst because this is a time of day when the participant may be fatigued, but it's also time for a shift in the daily activities.

When we were young, we got home from school at this time. As parents of school-aged children, we had to make sure we were home at this time to meet them. As a working adult, this often signaled the end of the shift and the time to go home. So the participant likely needs to shift gears to focus on a task reflective of where she is on her journey. You will need to listen to the concerns she expresses and address them correctly for the time period she is concerned about.

For instance, if she is concerned that she needs to get home for the children, ask her if the children would like to have some cookies and milk when they get home and if maybe you could bake some together. If she is in a period further back and is trying to get home to her parents, focus on a chore she can do for her mother.

Provide Opportunities Every Day to Share Successes. Seek Her Advice When Appropriate and Ask for Her Help.
A couple can talk about their wedding day or the birth of their children or how nervous they were on their first date, anything that stirs up a happy memory. Looking at photos together is a wonderful way to reminisce. As a daughter, you can talk about your childhood with your mother and share laughs and memories. If you don't have much personal history with the participant, you can still ask her about her wedding, her first date, and so on, and go that direction with the conversation. You can also seek her advice on areas in which she was knowledgeable. If you know she had a green thumb, ask for gardening advice; if she knows about the Bible, ask her questions about faith. If she was a teacher, solicit her advice about how to get kids to listen. Everyone has skills that they would love to share if asked! This is so important in stages 3 through 5 because participants have a sense of losing their identity and feelings of depression. So when you ask for advice, you will probably get good advice, and they will enjoy giving it.

Provide Regular Opportunities to Contribute to Others, Such as Volunteering at the Local Animal Shelter or Taking the Newspaper to the Shut-In Next Door
We all like to feel that we can still contribute, whether on a large or small scale, and feel as if we are part of something bigger than ourselves. If she knows someone needs her help or is counting on her, she will come through most every time and feel good about herself in the process. Focus on the things near to her heart and tailor them to her abilities so she can be successful. If you make a commitment to a charity to be there every

Thursday to feed all the animals, then you will have to be there every Thursday because they are counting on both of you. Most folks with dementia also struggle with depression. They have lost so much, and focusing on the needs of others goes a long way in helping improve mental health.

Ensure That Personal Care Is Attended To by Providing the Cues and Assistance Needed While Maintaining as Much Independence as Possible, Never Stealing Her Dignity
At first, the reminder notes or laying out of personal care items provided enough of a cue to get the task done, but as your loved one declines, more step-by-step instructions will be necessary. For instance, you are helping her put her slacks on and tell her to pick up her foot. She may not do it because she did not make sense of all of the words you were using so did not understand the instruction. The combination that would be most helpful here is to say, "Pick up this foot," and then tap the foot. If that doesn't work, place your palm just behind and above the knee and say, "Up." Once you have gotten the first leg done, she may respond more easily for the second. The key here is to use a combination of cues: verbal and physical or touch.

When you want your loved one to follow you to the bathroom, you may say, "Let's go to the bathroom," and then also make a gesture with your hand for her to come. This gives the brain two opportunities to understand what you are trying to communicate. If you want her to sit on the bed, but she doesn't understand, simplify it. Say, "Sit," and then pat the spot where you want her to sit.

When assisting with the shower once she is no longer able to take one independently, still give her as much autonomy as you can (you will probably want a shower seat and handheld sprayer if possible). For instance, put some soap on the washcloth for her to use and tell her you will wash her feet and her back while she washes the rest of her body. While you are doing that, you can see if she missed anything and just quickly go over those areas. And then let her rinse away. Generally two showers a week are sufficient for personal hygiene, but if she is in the habit of taking more, that's great. Showering may become more of an issue as the disease progresses, so don't worry about more than two a week if it causes conflict.

Some folks are frightened or scream when the water hits them. I believe it's because the stimulus is misinterpreted by the brain as a pain signal, which triggers a pain response of screaming or crying out. It may feel like hot, prickly water is hitting her. If that is the case for you, start the handheld sprayer at her feet and work your way up. If it is too much pressure on her skin, then hold the sprayer off to the side a little, and just use the washcloth on her body. She may be more comfortable in a bathtub, but most likely it will be too difficult to get her in and out of the tub, so the shower usually works the best.

Once your loved one starts having episodes of incontinence, you will have to be more active about personal hygiene. I prefer pull-up type disposable underwear. You will also want to purchase the disposable washcloths with the right pH balance for delicate skin. If she does a good job of getting herself clean, great, but you may want to assist in making sure.

Since she may not realize when she needs to go to the bathroom, you can follow this schedule of bathroom breaks to reduce the number of accidents: when she first gets up in the morning, a few minutes after breakfast, before and after lunch, before and after dinner, and before bed. If she wakes during the night, encourage her to go the bathroom then as well. Fidgeting with her belt or waistband or increased anxiety, wandering, or rubbing of her stomach may be signals that she needs to go to the bathroom.

Keep a Sense of Humor!

I would say that this, above all else, is most important. Your loved one is struggling. She may also realize that she is a burden on you and be trying hard to make sense of her environment. Dreams are intermingled with reality, and she is frustrated to say the least. When you acknowledge her frustration and do not add to it, you are building trust. Imagine yourself learning something new. You responded so much better to a teacher or coach who made it fun, and everyone laughed together and learned together. You are learning new skills and a new life as a caregiver, and your loved one is declining a little bit every day. Laughing together will make the journey more enjoyable.

8

Handling Sensitive Issues

Money

IN STAGE 4, you may want to consider giving her some cash (maybe fifteen to twenty dollars) to keep in her wallet with her identification and insurance cards but removing the credit cards and checkbook. Sometimes this is a sore subject, so try removing one card at a time. At the very least, make copies of all insurance cards, identification, and so forth, and store it in your wallet, with an additional copy someplace else. If you need to tell a little fib here, feel free to do so. You may tell her that you accidentally used the last check, so she will have to wait until the new ones arrive before spending any more money. This usually works and doesn't cause much grief, and it avoids perhaps a significant issue later with a large purchase or stolen account number.

Everyone's financial situation and vulnerability are different. Be aware that the participant may order items from an info-mercial or telephone solicitor, and any way you can delay her in completing a transaction will be helpful. For instance, you could keep the checkbook in a drawer away from the front door with a not attached to not give a check to anyone without calling you. However, you don't want to take away all her independence either. If she usually bought Girl Scout cookies, then let her buy them this year and have the satisfaction of helping the little girl down the street. Whether buying something for the baseball team fund raiser, supporting the local animal shelter, or putting an offering in the church basket, whatever is normal is fine. Just be on the lookout for unusual behavior or someone taking advantage.

Driving

It can be really hard to take the keys away from someone you know should not be driving. This is often the worst time for a family. You have several options, some less unpleasant than others, but you will likely have to be the bad guy. I'm sorry, but that's just the way it is. You are doing it for your loved one's safety and the safety of everyone else on the road. How would you feel if she caused an accident and killed someone when you knew that she shouldn't be driving but didn't have the backbone to do the right thing? You would never forgive yourself. Seek help from the doctor if your loved one will not agree that she shouldn't be driving. If the doctor says she shouldn't, then maybe she will remember and not try (not likely), but at least you can blame the doctor, and it won't be your fault she can't drive.

If you are concerned that she may still grab the keys and go, you must hide them or disable the car, and then you can lie about it.

"I don't know where the keys are. I'll look for them after dinner."

"I don't know what's wrong with the car. I'll look at it in a little bit."

You might disconnect the battery cable. You can also park the car somewhere else and claim it is in the shop. Whatever you have to say or do to keep her from driving is your responsibility to do. There is really no sugarcoating this.

Fortunately, many folks realize that they are not able to see as well as they used to or are not as comfortable driving in an unfamiliar area and will limit their driving on their own. Take this opportunity to take over and then just keep it up. Most states have a program that allows citizens to call in a complaint about someone who shouldn't be driving. The DMV will write a letter requiring that person to take a driver's test. Only do this if you are sure that your loved one will fail. Another option is to let her license expire for more than thirty days, by which time she will have to take the driver's test again. Then, if she fails, she won't have a license. Most seniors, when you remind them that they don't have a license, will not try to drive since they know it is wrong.

Getting Affairs in Order
Some paperwork will be needed when the time comes that your loved one is no longer competent to make her own decisions. You will need to speak with an attorney, preferably one who specializes in elder law, to complete these documents as soon as possible. Once she is deemed incompetent, it will be too late as she will not be able to make those decisions. She will most likely need a durable power of attorney and an advanced health-care directive, at the least. Depending on your family structure, the state you live in, and the amount of money she has, other options may also be appropriate. You must get legal advice and then discuss it with all family members involved in her care to make the best decision for your situation. Don't rely on the advice of friends, as their situations may be very different from yours.

Using Props
If you visit a memory care unit, you may see props dotted around the community such as a nursery, workbench, desk with supplies,

or perhaps a vanity with scarves, hats, and jewelry. These can be very valuable in turning around a difficult situation. For example, one resident used to wander through the halls nonstop for hours on end. One day, her daughter, Kelly, came in to visit her. It was Kelly's birthday, and she wanted to spend some time with her mom, walking alongside her. Kelly really wanted her mom to acknowledge that she was there but was not having any luck. I approached with a baby doll and commented on what a beautiful baby she was. The resident smiled widely and said, "Kelly is my beautiful baby," and cuddled the baby doll for a few steps before handing her back. Kelly had tears in her eyes. At that moment she knew her mother was remembering the bond between them when she was a baby. Buried treasure! It was a perfect birthday gift for her!

Baby dolls can also be utilized when the participant is stressed and fatigued. I have often asked a resident to please rock the baby for a few minutes. They almost always agree, rocking themselves to sleep in the process. The nurturing instinct is the last to go, and when nurturing another, we nurture ourselves.

Other props can be used to stimulate memories and start conversations. Sit at the vanity together and try on hats and boas. You'll likely be surprised at the stories you will hear! If she used to work in an office, ask her to work on some projects at the desk, such as clipping coupons, cutting out articles from the newspaper, or sorting the office supplies. These are all good tasks that will not only pass the time but give her a sense of fulfillment in work completed.

Many men of this generation did not have much time for hobbies such as golf and cards, so it can be difficult to engage them with leisure activities. All of their time may have been spent between work, chores, church, and sleep. The workbench can be very useful in simulating projects that you need his help with. The most successful have projects that appear to have been started, so he only needs to step up and continue working on them. It may be much harder to engage him if the items are not already laid out and ready to go. An unfinished project will draw him in. Again, it's important to praise and ask for advice on how it should be finished and so on, as the time spent working on the project together is very valuable in building trust.

9

Behavior Changes

Using the Bathroom

WE WANT TO do everything possible to keep the participant continent and using the bathroom as independently as she can for several reasons. It helps sustain her confidence and sense of independence, keeps the laundry workload at a reasonable level, and makes it easier to maintain good personal hygiene. There are a few things you can do to help remind and cue your loved one to use the bathroom.

First, encourage or remind her at the times we mentioned earlier—when she wakes up in the morning, after breakfast, before and after lunch, before and after dinner, and before bed. Usually about thirty minutes after a meal is when a bowel movement is most likely, so you don't want to miss that opportunity.

Second, you could install a motion sensor at the bathroom doorway and attach it to the light; when she walks by the bathroom the light will come on, giving her a gentle cue that she may need to use it.

Third, you may want to paint the wall behind the toilet a darker color, as this can help her distinguish the toilet from the other things in the bathroom and remind her to use it.

Fourth, we of course want to promote using the correct facilities, but we also need to discourage her from using inappropriate places. You may find that she goes into the den or office and uses the office chair or a vanity bench in the bedroom as a toilet. Other items commonly used are trash cans, plants, wall or space heaters, or even just a corner. The easiest thing to do is move the office chair or place it upside down on the desk when not in use and place trash cans under sinks or desks, not out in the open.

It is more common for men to use plants than women, so you may decide to just move them to a different part of the house. If you have wall-mounted heaters or space heaters, you may wish to put something in front of them, not so close as to be a fire hazard but close enough that the heater is not in the field of vision. The participant's brain sees the heater, but the brain misinterprets its function and believes it to be a toilet or urinal so the behavior makes perfect sense in his mind. A chair in front of the vanity may remind her of the bathroom, and so her using it as such is normal.

Lastly, if all of the above interventions are not successful and the participant is urinating in inappropriate places or out in public, you have the option of a clothing barrier. You may find that fastening her belt buckle in the back will prevent her from going to the bathroom without your help, eliminating the problem. Another option could be tying a knot in a scarf used as a belt. If these options no longer work, then a jumpsuit that zips up the back is the last resort. These can look like normal outfits from the front to maintain dignity, but they can only be removed with the help of someone else.

I'll admit, at first I was not comfortable with these tactics, but I realized over time that by saving someone from doing something embarrassing, I was preserving their dignity. That is very important in providing care in an honorable way.

Please try not to get angry with the participant. She is trying to be independent, and the behavior makes sense in her mind. She does not realize that she is doing anything wrong. Be sensitive to her feelings, and remember that sense of humor! However, it is up to you as the caregiver to alter the environment to reduce the chances that she will repeat the behavior.

Exit Seeking/Wandering

It is very common for a participant in stages 3 through 6 to wander or try to leave her home. Roughly half the folks with Alzheimer's dementia eventually wander. It may start suddenly without any warning; that is when the participant is most vulnerable to injury or prolonged exposure to the elements, falling victim to foul play, or even dying.

Wandering usually starts with a legitimate reason for leaving the house. She goes outside to check the mail or walk the dog. Somewhere along the way, she gets sidetracked, keeps walking, then later looks around and realizes that she is lost—or, worse, she just keeps walking, looking for something familiar but getting farther and farther from home.

If she encounters someone, she probably will not ask for help and may even refuse help if it is offered. To make matters worse, she may not be dressed for the weather. She also may not be as surefooted as she once was, and walking for a significant period of time, especially on uneven terrain, greatly increases her chance of falling and hurting herself.

She may also leave the home because she sees a car outside that she believes is her car or her ride to somewhere that she needs to go. This is more common in the afternoon sundowning period. If you can keep her busy then, doing a task that she believes needs to be done, she is less likely to be anxious and looking for the ride in the first place.

If the participant has wandered off and you find her after a search, it is important to approach her from the front and not from behind so as not to startle her. By the time you find her, she may be afraid and you don't want to add to that fear. If you don't find her within a few minutes, call family, friends, and neighbors to help you search familiar places or routes she may have taken. But don't wait too long to involve the police. They have a special alert they can broadcast to help with the search. The longer you wait, the larger the geographic area that must be searched. If your local police department has search and rescue dogs, they can smell an article of clothing from the home and follow the trail. If they are hours behind, however, your chances of finding her unharmed are greatly reduced.

The Alzheimer's Association also has a program called Safe Return. Please refer to their website to learn about it and any others that may be available in your area.

In an earlier section, we talked about using a door chime or door alarm to alert you when the door is open. If you haven't done that, please do that immediately, as you don't know when this behavior may start. If she has wandered off before and you haven't implemented any safety precautions, please put the book down and do so now.

The next line of defense is security locks. Be very careful here. I have seen deadbolt locks that require a key for both the outside and the inside installed on every door, with the keys kept away from the door in the interests of security. What if there was a fire, and no one could get out of the house? This is not a good solution. Since most folks with dementia primarily look at things at eye level, a deadbolt lock high or low on the door may be a better solution—one that can be unlocked from the inside without a key. The object here is not to lock the participant in but to alert caregivers that she is trying to open the door, and give them an opportunity to intervene.

In a care facility, the doors are secured, but they are also controlled by a sophisticated fire system, so if there is a fire the locks release. They also may have locks that will open if you push on a release bar for a certain period of time, while setting off an alarm to alert staff that someone is trying to exit; these are tested frequently to maintain safety. Even so, this is not something you can likely do in a private home.

Sexuality

The brain's frontal lobe, which controls impulses, is often impaired in Alzheimer's disease. As a result, the participant may respond sexually to something she sees or hears, make what she would have once considered an inappropriate remark, or make a pass at someone. This behavior may be very different from anything you have ever experienced from her, and it may be very upsetting. Please understand that these impulses themselves are not abnormal; her filter is just not working like it once did. The best you can do here is to try to keep the stimulation at bay. If it was a movie or TV show that initiated the inappropriate response, be more aware of what she is watching or listening to.

Sometimes when a caregiver provides personal care, the participant does not understand this as a basic hygiene service, misinterprets it as a sexual gesture, and responds accordingly. If the caregiver is her spouse, it may not feel unusual, but it may feel very inappropriate for a son or daughter who never experienced that response from a parent. Sometimes, just the personal care itself may cause the participant to assume a bond and that the care is being provided by a spouse, even when it is not. Wearing latex gloves and keeping the participant covered as much as possible maintains a more clinical and less personal environment and may help.

In a care facility, the staff is accustomed to these behaviors and learns how to best approach the participant to reduce them. No one is very comfortable with it, but everyone learns to make the best of it. Remember that sense of humor; the situation will be less embarrassing if you can joke about it a little.

Eating
Often if you ask the participant if she is hungry, she will say that she is not, even if she needs to eat. It's better to assume that she is hungry if it is mealtime and just know that she will likely eat when you serve her. The more you can utilize aromas to stimulate the appetite, the better. You can also talk about food before you sit down to eat.

As the disease progresses, it's better to cut up the meat before setting it in front of her to avoid the belittling experience of standing over her to cut it up at the table. Playing soft music during the meal can help to relax her mind a little so she can act more on instinct instead of wondering and asking what she should do with the fork.

Focus on serving her things that she likes and can eat easily. As eating gets more difficult, serve softer and sweeter foods, and don't worry as much about variety as giving her things that you know she will eat so she gets the calories she needs. You can always supplement with a Boost or Ensure nutrition drink if needed to get the appropriate vitamins. Mixing a nutrition drink with ice cream in the blender is very effective!

Try to keep her using utensils as long as possible, with you guiding the food to her mouth. The action of moving her hand toward her mouth stimulates digestive juices more so than when you feed her.

If it becomes difficult to keep her seated long enough to eat a meal, try finger foods that she can eat while mobile, such as a peanut butter sandwich or apple slices, something she can hold in one hand. You may also want to give her a drinking cup with a handle and maybe even a lid if she often spills her drinks. A clear lid works best, so she can judge how much is in the cup. Sometimes straws are easier to navigate, so try that next if she has trouble with the cup and tips it too far up.

Allow plenty of time for her to eat at her own pace and without rushing. If you have some place to go, try to start the meal earlier instead of trying to hurry through it, which will only add to her anxiety. If you need to feed her quickly, then give her something like a sandwich that she can eat with her hands. Eating will likely get messier as time goes on, so look for some adult bibs or clothing protectors to keep her clothes from becoming soiled and ruined, but don't stress over it or scold her for making a mess.

Some folks have the opposite issue and are hungry all the time, which can be even more difficult to manage. The brain does not receive the message the stomach is full, so she is constantly looking for something to eat. Another possibility is that she may be bored and looking for something to do, and we assume that she is looking for food. First, try to find things to do away from the kitchen and see if that resolves things. If not, just try to stay away from the kitchen as much as possible after a meal. You can also give her snacks that take a long time to eat but are still somewhat healthy, such as pistachios in the shell. After eating, go outside for a walk or work in the yard for a while to get her mind off eating.

In the worst-case scenario, if she is eating far too much, you may have to hide some food to keep her from eating too much junk and sugar.

Dressing

We already talked about showering and changing clothes in another section, so let's focus now on layering of clothes. This is very common, either because she is cold or just doesn't want to take clothes off, so she puts more clothes on top of what she is already wearing. For the most part, this is not a big deal—unless it is ninety degrees outside and she might get overheated. Let's say she has four layers on. Instead of trying to get three layers off at one time, work on the outer layer, and then work on the next outer layer about thirty minutes later, until you get her down to the one or two layers that seem sufficient.

Make sure that her clothing and shoes are in good repair and not rubbing or cutting into her skin. Uncomfortable clothes and tight shoes can cause behavior problems, so watch for those things. You may also find that she has a few favorite things that she wants to wear all the time. It may be easier to buy some duplicates instead of trying to get her to wear different things.

If you just lay out the clothes needed, she may be able to dress herself appropriately. Try to lay them out in the order she needs to put them on. If she is anxious when changing clothes, talk about something pleasant all the way through the process or sing a song together to keep her mind off it. It is also a good time to reminisce about your favorite Christmas or vacation. Just keep moving through the tasks without making any fuss, and she may just go along with you.

Communication

As time goes on, she will have more trouble understanding you and making herself understood. It is important to speak more slowly and use fewer words. If she doesn't hear you, use the same words or reduce the number of words when you repeat yourself, but don't change the words. For instance, if you first said, "Let's go outside and take the trash to the curb," and she didn't hear you, you could repeat with, "Outside and take trash."

When she is trying to communicate with you, she may interchange words when she is talking. We call this "word salad." Make eye contact with her and watch for other signals that may help you interpret what she is saying. Sometimes just nodding and smiling are enough for her to move on and keep the conversation going.

If she is upset or anxious, do not raise your voice. Just keep a mellow demeanor, as it will be easier for her to calm down if you are not getting agitated along with her. If she gets very upset and argumentative or aggressive, just get off the streetcar for a few minutes. When you return it likely will have blown over. Never argue—you will always lose!

Sleep

Sleep can become more fitful, or you may find her sleeping for a substantial part of the day. In the earlier stages, keeping her busy and physically active throughout the day will likely help her sleep, as she will be physically tired at night. If she dozes on and off all day, she may have more trouble staying asleep at night.

There can also be a reason why she is not sleeping at night, and you will need to put on your detective hat to figure out what it is. I took care of a resident who wandered all evening while muttering numbers. He would get so sleepy that he would almost fall over, and we would get him to bed for a little while. Then he would be up an hour later, pacing and mumbling for hours on end. It was horrible for him and also would have likely led to a bad fall from exhaustion.

I spoke with some family members and learned that he used to be a switchman for the railroad. That night I asked him if he was calling the railcars in the yard, and he responded with an exasperated "Yes!" I told him that his replacement was now on duty, so he was off the clock and could rest. He was so relieved that he was able to sleep for several hours. Each time he woke up, and every night after that, we repeated that he was off the clock and the other switchman was in charge so that he would relax and go to sleep. This was buried treasure; there was a perfectly reasonable explanation for what he was doing and a very good solution to fix the behavior. A good day!

Some folks wander all night long for no underlying reason that you can ascertain. This can be very difficult if you are the only caregiver, as you cannot get your rest if you have one eye and ear open all night listening for her. This is often the last straw for a spouse who cannot get his rest, prompting placement in long-term care. Be sure to speak with the doctor about it, as there may be a medication that will work to help her sleep, but for some it doesn't help at all.

10

Psychiatric Issues

PSYCHIATRIC ISSUES IN Alzheimer's disease are often not spoken of until the problem is significant. As a caregiver, you may not understand what is going on and undergo significant verbal and physical abuse, embarrassment, and shame just because you didn't know how to respond to these issues or realize that they are not uncommon and seek the help you both needed.

For some folks the psychiatric issues start in stage 4 but are more often prevalent in stages 5 and 6. They can range from mild depression to severe paranoia and can include auditory and visual hallucinations and personality changes. Let's break it down to make some sense of how and why these things occur.

Alzheimer's disease ravages the brain, shrinking it over time and carving out holes so it looks like swiss cheese. Brain signals are not transmitted correctly along the normal pathways because of these gaps. If you remember when you were immersed in the story of a lady living alone, you were most confused when you first woke up. After you had some time to gather your thoughts and reconnect with your surroundings, you were able to remember things and function a little better. As a participant progresses through the stages of Alzheimer's, this reconnecting takes longer and longer until she reaches a point when she can't connect the dots anymore. I also believe that a person's personality traits will be exacerbated as the disease progresses. For instance, a person who would have been considered very moody in earlier years may have more dramatic mood swings as she progresses; someone who was considered obsessive about details will become even more so, and someone who was emotionally high strung could become extremely difficult as she declines.

We talked in an earlier chapter of the time-warp sensation of waking up and seeing nothing familiar. Imagine the horrible feeling of not being able to make any sense of your world, easy to understand why the participant may believe you are stealing all of her money; she may want you out of her house because she doesn't remember you are a family member. She may know your name when she looks at an old picture of you and know the relationship she has with you but does not realize that you are that same person forty years on.

This paranoia can be heightened if she intermingles dreams with reality. The brain tries very hard to make sense of its surroundings, so often the participant will believe that things she only dreamed about are true, or she may be unable to distinguish between her dreams and reality. She may be extremely aggressive toward you or resistant to your efforts to help her just because she can't make sense of her world.

Hallucinations, either auditory or visual, are virtually the same as dreams; they just happen when the participant is awake. If she is having a hallucination while you are there, do not tell her that it's not real. It will only cause her to distrust you. Instead, focus on whether the hallucination is causing her anxiety or bringing comfort. Sometimes if she is hallucinating about a spouse (who is deceased), it may bring her comfort to believe her husband is across the room talking to her. Just go along with it and reminisce or tell her he must be a wonderful husband. If the hallucination is causing anxiety, then take her out of the room to get away or try to distract her with something else. For instance, if she sees spiders on the wall, you could ask her where the spiders are and then say, "Let's get away from those spiders," and leave the room or go to a different area. Be sure to mention this to the doctor, and make a note of when these things happen to see if there is any pattern, as medications may help.

Mood swings or dramatic reactions to normal events can also lead to very difficult behavior. When you notice a significant mood swing, jot down what you were doing or talking about just before it happened, and watch for patterns so you can avoid the trigger in the future. Someone who always had a take-charge personality or liked to be in control is going to have a very difficult time with dementia, and you will likely take the brunt of her aggression when she knows she is losing control. As much as you can, make things seem like her idea, giving her choices throughout the day. Don't act like you are the boss. This will make things easier to manage.

A milder but often embarrassing change is the loss of the filter in the brain that tells us we shouldn't say something. Whatever she thinks, she will say, and these things can be hurtful to those closest to her. A person who never said a swear word may now "cuss like a sailor." Also, she may make racist or condescending remarks to complete strangers, making going out in public difficult. She may not hesitate to tell you that you are fat or that your haircut is not becoming or that your husband will never amount to anything. Sometimes these are legitimate observations that would have been better left unsaid, but sometimes they reflect underlying fears. She may have been afraid that your husband wouldn't amount to anything and be able to provide you with the lifestyle she wanted for you. It doesn't mean that she ever truly believed it, and it doesn't account for the twenty-five years you've been together or that he was a good husband, because she doesn't remember the twenty-five years, only the underlying fear when you were dating.

The good news is that medications can really help. It is so important to work with a physician who really understands Alzheimer's and can recommend and monitor medications. An in-patient geriatric psychiatric hospital may also be able to help if your loved one's behavior is just not manageable. It is very common for patients to need this type of in-patient treatment, and the medical staff and social workers will help you to handle the situation when she is discharged. Do not hesitate to ask your doctor about this wonderful option if you cannot manage the behavior on your own. As difficult as the behavior is on the outside, imagine the utter hell her mind must be in to cause her to act in that way. You have to get her some help.

It is not uncommon for the participant to complain of people hitting her, being mean to her, raping her, and so on. Such complaints are very hard to hear because you are of course concerned at first that they are true. It is almost worse to learn that the complaint is not true. Now you have to navigate those waters with the participant believing it is true and being angry with you if you don't believe it.

You will have to try some different things here to see which approach will work. There are entire books on validation therapy, so I will just touch on this. I was once caring for a lady who reported to me that one of the male aides had raped her the night before. She was frightened and angry and retold the story several times throughout the morning with perfect recollection. (Often memories, dreams, or hallucinations that are tied to an emotion, such as fear or anger, can be remembered in vivid detail.) I fuddled around all morning and did not handle it properly, only increasing her fear and indignation. I called her son and relayed the story that she had told. He told me that he had every confidence that the male aide had not done anything wrong, as she told this story every time he went out of town. So when she brought it up again a few hours later, I took her hands and looked in her eyes and expressed my horror at what had happened to her. I told her I knew she must have been very frightened and promised that I would not let anything happen to her ever again.

When the male aide came in that afternoon for his shift, she started telling her story again and was very angry. I took her hands and told her that she was safe now, and we walked out of the room and away from the aide. I scheduled another aide to care for her the rest of the week, and anytime she brought it up, we just continued to tell her that she was safe now and that we wouldn't let anything happen to her. As the days went on, we never told her it didn't happen and never treated it as a bad dream. We just focused on calming her fears and promising to keep her safe. When her son returned from his trip, she stopped telling the story. She felt vulnerable when he was away, and that manifested itself into a vivid, frightening dream that became her reality.

11

Caregiver Issues

How Long Should You Continue Taking Her with You on Errands?

THIS WILL OF course vary by situation, but structure and routine are very important, and when you control the environment, you can protect her better. When you are out in the car and in public, there are many variables outside of your control. Usually when the participant is in stage 4 or early in stage 5, errands are fine for shorter periods of time; just don't let her get overtired. If you are taking her to day care, you can continue that as long as she is getting benefit from it, as the staff there will be trained in how to best interact with her. However, going with you to several stores and interacting with numerous people who don't know her could certainly cause significant anxiety in some, while others will go along just fine for months or years but have a catastrophic reaction one day to a loud noise or a car horn. You just never know, so watch for signs of stress and be ready to adjust your plans quickly. If you have child locks on your car doors and are at all concerned that she may try to get out of the moving car, put her in the backseat.

When Is It Time to Consider a LTC (Long-Term Care) Solution?

Usually the answer is sooner than later. At least consider that you may not be able to handle this alone, and take the time to explore options in your community before you need them. I have mostly spoken of the caregiver as the spouse and being there full time because presumably he is retired. This is feasible, but for other family members trying to provide full-time care, it may be more difficult, as there are others in the picture. For instance, her daughter may have children at home who need her attention or may be working full time; a niece or nephew may be willing to participate in caregiving decision making but unable to provide hands-on supervision.

Remember imagining that you live alone? In the absence of a spouse, perhaps someone visiting a couple of times a day and spending some time with you would fill the gap. A neighbor, family member, or hired companion could visit for an hour or two a couple of times a day to make sure you take your medicine, eat a healthy meal, get some exercise, and help you with household tasks. This may be just enough support for months or even a couple of years. As a participant declines, an extra visit or extending the visits may be necessary but still enough to keep her in her home. Adding in adult day care would be very beneficial as well. However, if she starts to wander, then she is no longer safe alone and would then have to have a family member move in with her or her with them, hire full-time caregivers, or move into a memory care community. These would be the only safe solutions at that point.

You Need a Break.
Even when a spouse is the primary caregiver, extra help for a few hours a day every day or a few hours a couple of days a week can tip the balance in favor of being able to provide care at home for a much longer time. This help could be a volunteer, neighbor, friend, family member, or hired companion. Be very careful when hiring someone you do not know and paying him or her directly. Whomever you hire will be alone in your home and alone with your loved one, who will likely not be able to

tell you if he or she was snooping through your things, and so forth. You probably don't have the resources to do a proper background screen and reference check.

Even someone who is totally trustworthy may get injured while working in your home. Some homeowners' policies do not cover hired help, and you would then be on the hook for the medical expenses. Even though it may seem more expensive, it usually makes sense to hire an agency that specializes in caring for those with memory loss. Make sure the agency is insured, carries workman's compensation on their employees, does background screenings, and provides regular staff training and oversight. Ask around for recommendations, and then interview two or three agencies to make sure you are making a good choice. If the agency will let you select the companion, that's even better.

In stages 3 through 6, adult day care is a good option if there is one close by; some even provide transportation. If she spends eight hours a day there, two to five days per week, she will have socialization, activities, assistance with personal care, and maybe nursing supervision. If the spouse is the primary caregiver, this can provide a significant break for him to enjoy other hobbies and have a break from caregiving. It is more cost effective than agency companions, and your plans are not contingent on whether the home-care worker shows up on a given day! It is also great for the caregiver who is still working, as day programs are designed to meet the needs of the working caregiver as well.

Everyone has his or her limits as a caregiver, and hopefully the information provided in this book will make your task seem more manageable. But even with knowledge, skills, and passion, you may not be physically able to do it. Financial constraints may prevent you from providing the needed day-to-day oversight. Perhaps you are still working and not able to afford a companion to stay with your wife while you are at work. Or your own health concerns may mean you are not able to handle the stress and physical requirements of full-time caregiving. That is OK! *Do not lose any sleep over guilt!*

Remember how I said it takes a village? Well, it's time to utilize that village. She still needs you to be her caregiver, but you don't have to be the one providing continuous oversight. You still will have important decisions to make; you are the one making sure that she is as happy and content as possible and overseeing her medical care. You are a vital part of her well-being.

I'll be honest with you—many folks can handle the full-time caregiving as long as their loved one is continent. But once those accidents start and the laundry workload increases significantly as well as the effort to keep the participant clean and dry—or when they can't get her to take a needed shower—the task becomes overwhelming. This is often when people realize they can't do it anymore.

There are some definite advantages to moving your loved one to a memory care facility. She will have instant friends with whom she can share her day without feeling judged or unable to keep up, and she will have assistance with her personal care without feeling guilty that you are the one providing it. She will have many new things to do that she will enjoy, and she will have numerous opportunities to be successful throughout the day—things that you never thought of. She will be happy to see you when you visit, and after she settles in, she will also be ready for you to leave so she can resume her activities. She will have a sense of purpose in her day, as many people are counting on her to join in—there is peer pressure on residents to get involved and be more active. It will be easier for you to adjust if you realize that no matter how good a job you did as a primary caregiver, you are only one person, and now she has a "village"—not only the staff but her new friends as well.

You will want to look for a place that specializes in dementia, whether it is a nursing home or a memory care assisted living center. You can search online or use a service, such as A Place for Mom, to help you find one. On the Medicare.gov website, you can search for nursing homes, but they don't currently rank assisted living communities.

Once you select one, follow their guidance on whether you should visit in the first few days; sometimes it is helpful to stay away and let her adjust to her new surroundings. If you choose this path, then feel free to call and check on her each day. In my experience, it seems best to stay away for a couple of days and then visit about an hour before a meal. At that point, you can walk her to the dining room and slip away while she is visiting with her tablemates. Out of sight is out of mind, and you'll avoid a big scene should she want to leave with you.

If she complains to you that people are not taking care of her, she is not eating, and so forth, be wary. You will want to investigate, but also realize that just because she may not remember that she ate doesn't mean that she didn't. Use your best judgment, and give the staff the benefit of the doubt until you have a reason not to. Watch for significant weight loss, abnormal bruising, and so forth, but mostly watch how she responds to the staff. If she seems comfortable with them, then most likely they are providing good care. No place is perfect. They will make mistakes or not do something the way you think it should be done, but try to keep an open mind and remember how hard it was for you to care for her. Realize that the staff have significantly more residents to care for and that they are doing their best. Of course, if there is a problem, don't hesitate to speak up quickly and often until it is resolved; if you are not satisfied with her care, look elsewhere.

12

Hospice

HOSPICE CARE FOR end of life is currently covered by Medicare and insurance companies. Since AD is a fatal disease, participants are generally eligible for hospice when they meet certain criteria, usually significant weight loss, frequent infections, or frequent falls. It is available wherever the participant lives and provides care and support for both the participant and the family. Generally a nurse will visit one to two times per week, and a bath aide will visit two to three times per week to assist with personal care. A chaplain and social worker also visit regularly to provide support. Some previously out-of-pocket costs may be covered by hospice, such as some medications and incontinence products, as well as any medical equipment needed, such as a hospital bed, wheelchair, Hoyer lift, and so on. As she declines, more help will be brought in to meet her needs and keep her comfortable; however, the primary tasks still reside with the family or care center, as the hospice staff only provides services while they are there for a "visit." Once a patient is considered "actively dying," hospice may provide constant care or come every few hours to make sure the patient is comfortable, but agencies can vary on this. You will want to interview at least two agencies and get recommendations from others before choosing one. Select one that truly understands dementia and will be respectful of your loved one's needs as well as yours.

Get out the *Caring Conversations* booklet and share it with the hospice personnel so that they can truly understand what your loved one wants and honor those wishes. If for any reason you do not believe that they will be willing to do so, then select another agency.

End of Life

There are of course the physical or medical conditions that one expects at the end of life. But it is the spiritual and emotional ones that will have the most impact as you end this journey with your loved one. This is where the knowledge, skills, and passion you poured into caregiving will come full circle.

As her body shuts down and troubled sleep engulfs her day, you will provide the sensory experiences to reduce her anxiety that you mastered over the previous months. Her faith may be strong, but fear of the unknown can also be overwhelming, especially if she is struggling to interpret your words. She may need permission to let go or need to hear from family members through visits or phone calls. You need to make sure she is given that opportunity. I have sat with many folks as they took that last breath, and it is remarkably joyous when you know that you did your best to care for them, have kept them comfortable through their last days, and have spared them unnecessary anxiety.

"You never know how strong you are until being strong is the only choice you have."

—Bob Marley

One lady I helped care for seemed to hang on for days in a mostly comatose state. All of her family had visited and said their good-byes. Those who couldn't visit had called on the phone, and we put the phone to her ear—sometimes she seemed to recognize them, but she said nothing and didn't even open her eyes. After two more days, I remembered her love of music and dancing and asked some ladies to come in and sing an upbeat song that she would have danced to if she were able. They obliged, and all had tears streaming down their faces as she moved one finger to the beat of their music. She passed away a few minutes later, dancing all the way to heaven. Buried treasure—my final gift to her.

Appendix

MEMORY/PROJECT STATIONS, use what you feel most appropriate

- Jigsaw puzzle, one hundred pieces (reduce if it becomes too challenging)
- Basket of unsorted socks
- Basket of unmatched earrings
- Basket of towels to be folded (love this one)
- Wedding album, baby books
- Nuts, screws, bolts that can be sorted
- Coupons that need to be cut out
- Cookbooks to look through
- Scrapbook, memory box that has been completed
- Junk mail to be sorted
- Business cards to be alphabetized
- Dishes to be hand-washed
- Scrabble pieces—make smaller words with the letters
- Word searches
- Button basket—sort by color
- Hobby basket—items used in former hobby (e.g., golf tees, balls, ball marker, golf towel, pictures, golf spikes, score cards) he can rummage through and reminisce about

- Nursery basket—baby items such as bottle, pacifier, socks, sleepwear, hats, baby soap (for the fragrance), blanket, and so forth as a reminder of happy times
- Scents to smell and talk about
- Deck of cards to sort by color
- Occupation basket—items used in a former occupation (e.g., calculator, pencil, graph paper, envelopes, stamps, etc.)
- Sports basket—items from high school or college sports, or memorabilia from favorite sports teams

www.ingramcontent.com/pod-product-compliance
Lightning Source LLC
Chambersburg PA
CBHW070934180526
45168CB00003B/1070